Heal Your Body, Live Your Life!

Heal Your Body, Live Your Life!

Healing lower back pain without medicine, shots or surgery

Dr. Sara S. Morrison

ISBN: 1540485986
ISBN 13: 9781540485984

This book is dedicated to:
My husband Erik, for his never ending love, support and ability to make me laugh!
My mother, for showing me how to be a strong, compassionate and loving woman
And most of all, my son Blake Patrick. You are the light of my life!

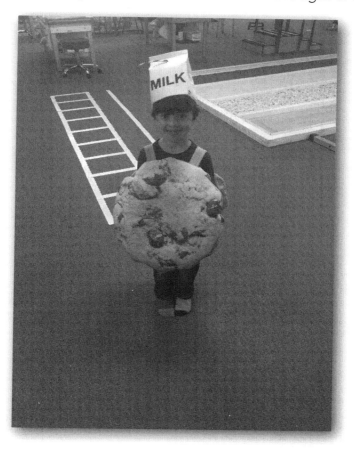

Table of Contents

Forward

Do you have lower back pain?
Are you tired of missing work, missing out on family activities or even missing sleep because of your pain?
Do you want to feel better WITHOUT medication, shots or surgery???
Then this book is for YOU! I am here to tell you it is possible to "Heal Your Body, Live Your Life!" naturally, safely and effectively.

OVER THE YEARS I have found it increasing hard for people to find accurate information on healing their pain. Sure, there is a ton of information out there! Just search "back pain" on the internet and thousands upon thousands of sites will come up. But is it accurate? Can you really believe it? Much of it is misleading. It is someone trying to sell you something. Others are just plain wrong! So how is a non-medical person supposed to find accurate information on improving their pain? That is why I wrote this book. I hope you enjoy it.

And if you like it, please share it with a friend.

I graduated from PT school in 2002 and I headed South. I always wanted to live in the sunshine by the beach. The plan was for my husband (fiancé at the time) and I to move to Virginia Beach for about 2 years, get some experience, and then move back to

Western New York. I was going to get a job at the local hospital, have my 2.5 kids and lead a quiet life.

But that was not God's plan for me.

As I continued looking for jobs I found myself falling in love with North Carolina. I had 1 interview there… it was a horrible job… but I LOVED the area! So I changed my target to NC. One hot Summer day, I found myself in Harnett County in a small waiting room. I was a 21 year old girl, far away from home, nervous and sweating in my heavy black suit. As I was waiting for my interview, several of the patients in the waiting room began talking to me. They were so friendly and genuine. They eased my nerves helped me relax. When I walked off to my interview they even hugged me and wished me good luck! Something told me I had just found my new home… and the interview had not even begun! It turns out my husband had a very similar experience talking to people at the gas station as he waited for me. We both knew Harnett County was where we belonged! As time went on, we continued to fall in love with North Carolina, the people, the strong family values … and of course… the sun!

Several years after living in North Carolina I lost my job. I literally walked up to find the Sheriff locking the door. "Don't bother" he said "This place is closed". I came home sad and afraid. We were barely making ends meet as it was. What about my patients? Where would they go? I knew they would not travel to Raleigh or Fayetteville for care. Most people would just go on hurting. I didn't want that to happen. It was then that my husband convinced me to open my own clinic. He helped me remember my frustrations about not being able to treat my patients the way I wanted. This would give me the opportunity to do that! With his unending support and encouragement, I opened Total Body Therapy & Wellness in July of 2008. My plan was to operate this by myself for 6 months or a year. By then I would hopefully have enough money to hire an office person. My long term goal, in my wildest dreams, was that I would one day have enough need for a Rehab Technician, an office person and maybe, just maybe, a PT Assistant.

Yet again, the Big Man upstairs had other plans.

Within 3 months I was hiring a receptionist and by a year or so I had my first PT Assistant and 2 Rehab Technicians. By treating people the way I wanted to treat them… with Hands-On or Manual style therapy, love and compassion… my business exploded! People may not know about physical therapy, or even health care, but they know when they are being treated right. And they spread the word.

Never in a million years did I think I would own my own business. Let alone have 20+ employees, win a Small Business of the Year award, be the President of the Lillington Chamber of Commerce, conduct interviews for prospective Doctorate of Physical Therapy students at Campbell University or speak at dozens of community events and groups every year! God's plan is often different from our own. I thank him for always putting me in the right situation to better follow His plan. Through the years I have had many trials and tribulations, but He always provides me with what I need, not what I want, at the exact time I need it. He has put me here to help the people of Harnett County heal … and I have loved every minute of it!

I hope you enjoy this book. I want everyone to be able to "Heal Your Body, Live Your Life!"

— *Sara*

1

What's Wrong with my Back??

THERE ARE SEVERAL ways to diagnose lower back pain. The first step is your history. Your health care provider will ask you questions on when and how your back pain started, where it is located and what it feels like. They will also ask you when it occurs. It is important to mention if you have had a recent injury, such as a fall, car accident, collision or any type of a trauma. Here are some questions your provider may ask you:

1. When did the pain start?
2. Was there any type of injury?
3. Where is the pain located?
4. How strong is the pain on a scale from 0-10? (both at the best and at worst)
5. What makes the pain worse?
6. What makes the pain feel better?
7. Have you tried to do anything for the pain? If so, what?

When you are preparing to speak with your provider, it is a good idea to think about the answers to these questions in advance.

From that information your provider will decide if imaging is necessary. These images can include:

1. X-ray
    a. This shows the bones and their alignment. This is useful for seeing things such as breaks, fractures, arthritis and alignment or position of the bones.
    b. These are very cheap, quick and easy to perform, but are much more limited in what they can show
2. MRI (Magnetic Resonance Imaging)
    a. This shows a much more in depth picture of all the tissues in the body. This includes discs, tendons, muscles, tears, nerves and even swelling.
    b. In MRI the bones do not affect the images of organs or soft tissues, so they may be used instead of computed tomography (CT) when organs or soft tissue are being studied.
    c. Because radiation is not used, there is no risk of exposure to radiation during an MRI procedure.
    d. MRI's cannot be used over an area that has metal (screws, plates, shrapnel, etc).
3. CT Scan (Computerized Axial Tomography Scan)
    a. This can show anything that is bad, including, tumors, ulcers, cancer etc in more detail than an MRI. People often have CT scans to further evaluate an abnormality seen on another test such as an X-ray, MRI or an ultrasound
    b. The CT scan uses radiation, just like an x-ray
    c. Can be used as an alternative to MRI if you have metal in the area.

If you have not had an injury, trauma or fall, imaging is not required to begin treatment. If no trauma has occurred, you can proceed directly to a physical therapist without going to the doctor.

Evaluation

There are several steps to an evaluation for lower back pain. After questions your PT will closely examine your body. They will measure how far you can move in each direction. They will also assess how your back, hips and legs stretch. They will examine your posture, and feel your back and hips for tender areas, soreness, swelling, pain points and muscle abnormalities. These include atrophy (where the muscle is wasted away or smaller), spasms (where the muscles are very tight) or knots. You will then go through what we call Special Tests. These are different positions and activities that can assess what is wrong with your body without scans (x-ray, MRI, CT, etc). The therapist will have you move certain ways, stretch your body in various directions or have you try to perform certain movements to accurately assess the injury. Contrary to popular belief, we do not enjoy making you hurt! (Well, maybe a little…) Unfortunately the best way to find out what is wrong is to find out what makes you hurt. Painful activities, positions and areas on the body will give your therapist good information on what is wrong. It's much cheaper than those other tests!

There are 4 main issues you can have with your back:

1. Bulging/ Herniated Disc
2. Arthritis or Degeneration
3. Sacro-Iliac Dysfunction
4. Posture

2

Bulging or Herniated Disc

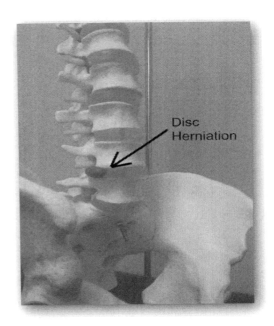

Disc
Herniation

THE DISCS ARE the cushions of your spine that are between each bone or vertebrae. Each disc has a firmer outside with a jelly-like inside. They are much like Jelly donuts. I call it the Homer Simpson theory. If you squeeze one end of the jelly donut, what happens?

The jelly comes out the opposite end. The same happens with our discs. When there is too much pressure on one side of the spine it will force the "jelly", or annulus, out of the other side. This is referred to as a "bulging disc". Now, if you take that same jelly donut and squeeze harder, what happens then? The jelly not only pushes out, but it leaks further outside the donut making a little circle of jelly. With your discs, when the annulus material is forced further outside the disc and makes this "puddle" it is called a "Protruding Disc".

Now I'm sure some of you don't like jelly donuts. (I prefer chocolate frosted myself) Let's say you don't want that donut and you stomp on it. What happens then? The jelly just shoots out of that donut and makes a mess all over the floor. (You also may be kicked out of that donut store).

In your spine this is called a Herniated Disc. This is when the force on your spine is so strong that the annulus material in your disc is exploded out of the outer edge of the disc. As you can imagine, this usually occurs with some kind of accident, fall or other injury.

The levels of disc injuries are measured by how far the annulus material is extended beyond the borders of the disc. One would think the more the disc is bulging or protruding the more painful the injury, but this is not so. You can take 2 MRI's on 2 different people, both with the same level of disc bulge, and they will have 2 different pain levels. Person #1 may feel horrible pain while person #2 does not have any symptoms. Therefore just because something shows up on an MRI or other scan, doesn't mean it's the issue that is causing pain. Along the same lines, the level of disc bulge does not always depict whether the person will require surgery or whether physical therapy will be enough to resolve the symptoms. For these reasons, MRI's are not always required. Most doctors suggest you try PT for 1 month and then reassess your symptoms before ordering an MRI. This saves you and your insurance company time and money on unnecessary testing.

I have 2 examples that illustrate this point:

1. I had one patient that had horrible pain in his back and shooting down his leg. He received an MRI which showed a bulging disc. This person was set up for surgery. A few days before surgery he found blisters along his trunk. It turned out that the pain in his back was really the Shingles and nothing to do with the bulging disc in his back. And he almost had unnecessary surgery!
2. I had another patient with a similar story. She had horrible pain in the back and leg. The MRI of her back showed Degenerative Disc Disease. This woman had surgery but no relief of her pain. She went back to the surgeon and he said everything was fine with the surgery. She went to several other specialists and one of them finally took an X-ray of her hip. It turns out that she had "bone-on-bone" in her hip joint. She needed a hip replacement… immediately… as in yesterday. It turns out, she never even needed that back surgery!

So, who cares if my jelly is leaking out of my donut??
(Well, first of all, we don't want to waste food…)

When the annulus or jelly pushes out of the disc it can press on the nerves. When the nerve gets pinched you can get that numb, tingling or burning feeling. You may also feel coldness, heat, aching or heaviness. The more the nerve is pinched, the farther this feeling will shoot. It can shoot into your hip, groin or all the way into your toes. If you feel your back pain shoot into your buttock, that means the nerve is getting pressed. If you bend over and the feeling shoots into your knee, that means that the nerve is getting pinched harder. In other words, when you feel the pain shoot farther STOP WHAT YOU ARE DOING! That means you are making it worse.

With therapy we are trying to accomplish 3 things:

1. The pain does not hurt as bad
2. The pain does not occur as often
3. The pain does not shoot as far

In my experience, when you have pain shooting or radiating down your leg, the FIRST sign that you are getting better will usually be #3, the pain does not shoot as far down your leg. It may hurt just as bad and it may occur just as often, but it will not shoot as far. This is an improvement. It can be frustrating as obviously everyone would rather it just not hurt as bad. But patience is a virtue and we do not always get what we want. Doing things the right way is not always fast. But if you really want to get better, and you want it to last, this is what you need to do.

So how do I know if I have a herniated or bulging disc?

1. You are under 35 years old
2. You have had a major injury, trauma or fall.
    a. Usually people know exactly when and how they got hurt
    b. Did you hear a "pop" when you got hurt?
    c. Can you tell me the exact moment you began hurting?
3. It hurts worse with sitting and bending forward
4. It feels better with standing

Pain is worse with:

1. Bending
2. Squatting
3. Lifting
4. Twisting
5. Sitting long periods
6. Driving/riding in vehicles
7. Coughing or sneezing

Pain is BETTER with:

1. Standing
2. Walking
3. Laying down

When you stand, your weight is distributed throughout your back and your legs. When you sit all of your weight is on your back and your spine. So if your problem is inside your spine it will hurt more with sitting. When you bend forward your vertebrae or bones in your spine squeeze the front part of your disc. This pushes the jelly backwards and worsens the bulge. Any time your body bends forward this will happen. Activities like bending, squatting, lifting and sitting for longer periods of time will often aggravate the pain. Activities that combine forward bending position with impact or bumping, such as driving in a car or riding a lawn mower, will be even worse for the pain. Pain is usually sharp and runs specifically down the back of the leg, possibly into the foot.

Hands on physical therapy can help put the "jelly" back in your "donut". By using the correct exercises we can force the disc to be in the proper spot and take pressure of your nerves (yay!) Physical therapists specialize in how to do this without aggravating your pain... and doing it without medication, shots, or surgery!

Once you can move with less pain we work on building your strength. When your muscles are strong, they can take the pressure off your spine and allow you to bend, move and do all your activities with less pain (double yay!) So what are you waiting for? Are you ready to "Heal Your Body, Live Your Life!" ??? Ask your PT about Hands-on or Manual physical therapy today!

3

Arthritis/ Degeneration

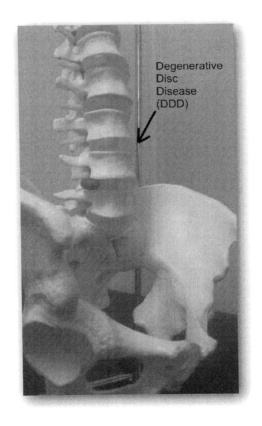

Degenerative
Disc
Disease
(DDD)

YOUR SPINE IS made up of bones (vertebrae) stacked on top of each other with discs in between each bone. Between each bone is a nerve running out the right and left sides. These nerves run from the back all the way down the leg into the toes. As we age degeneration or "wear and tear" is normal. In fact EVERYONE over the age of 50 will have some sort of degeneration in their spine, whether or not they have pain. This is normal after using your body year after year. As your body ages, you can have degeneration in your bones or your discs. When the bone degenerates it becomes shorter, known as Degenerative Joint Disease (DJD). When the discs degenerate they lose their fluid and also become shorter. This is known as Degenerative Disc Disease (DDD). Either way, the spine is now more compressed. You may notice you are not as tall as you once were. As the spine compresses there is less room for the nerves as they exit the spine. The holes the nerves travel out of become smaller and they are more likely to get pinched when you move. When you move the bones will slide and may pinch the nerve. This can cause pain in your back and shoot down the leg. The harder the nerves are pinched, the farther the pain will shoot. It can shoot into your hip, groin or toes. You may also feel numbness, tingling, burning, heaviness or cold sensations.

What makes me more likely to get arthritis?

1. Genetics
2. Trauma or Accidents earlier in life
3. Previous surgery in the area
4. Increases with age

DR. SARA S. MORRISON

How do I know if I have arthritis or Degeneration?

1. You had more than 50 candles on your last Birthday Cake
2. Achy, throbbing pain

Pain is WORSE with:

1. Walking
2. Standing
3. Damp, cold or rainy weather

Pain is BETTER with:

1. Sitting
2. Bending forwards

When you have arthritis, exercise is like greasing a wheel. At first it takes more effort to start, but after a while, it makes it much easier to move. By using the correct exercises and Hands-On, Manual style physical therapy, PT's can help you move better with less pain. Physical therapists specialize in how to do this without aggravating your pain... and doing it without medication, shots, or surgery!

Once you can move with less pain we work on building your strength. When your muscles are strong, they can take the pressure off your spine and allow you to bend, move and do all your activities with less pain (yay!) So what are you waiting for? Are you ready to "Heal Your Body, Live Your Life!" ??? Ask your PT about Hands-on or Manual physical therapy today!

4

Sacro Iliac Dysfunction (SIJ)

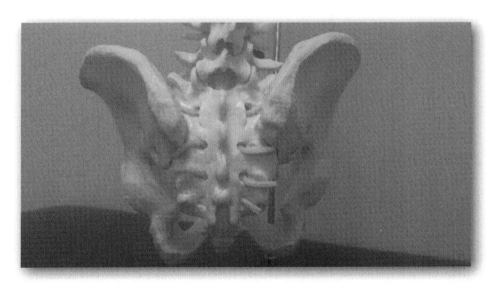

THE SACRUM IS a large upside down triangle shaped bone at the bottom of your spine. It is located at the top of your rear end. On each side of the sacrum is one of your pelvic bones, known as Iliac bones. The iliac bones are located next to the sacrum making up your Sacral-Iliac Joint or more commonly known as SIJ. This joint is not as secure as the other joints in your body. Take the hip joint for example. In the hip, the pelvic bone forms a cup and the thigh bone (Femur) fits right into the cup. In the hip joint the bones hold the joint securely. This is not the case with the SIJ as the bones "lay next to" each other instead of "fit inside" each other. This makes the SIJ much more easily injured. When the SIJ is involved it will cause pain with prolonged positions… such as remaining sitting over 15 or 20 minutes, or standing in one spot. It feels better with movement, especially walking.

The SIJ is usually injured in a 1-sided injury. This means that there was something that impacted one side more than another. This can be from a fall, a car accident (especially if one leg was bent more than another when you were hit) or something as simple as stepping down hard from a curb.

My clinic is located just North of Fort Bragg Military Base where they have a large Airborne division. I see many military members with SIJ issues after Airborne operations (aka- jumping out of a perfectly good airplane hundreds of feet above the ground. It's usually the "landing" part that causes the pain). The SIJ is an equal opportunity pain. It has equal chance of hitting men and women, young and old.

We all have been walking in the yard before and not seen a hole. If one foot was to step in a hole unexpectedly, the force will travel up your leg, thigh and impact at your pelvis. It can shift the iliac bone so that it is turned or rotated. With this type of injury most people do not realize that they have injured themselves. As time goes on, the muscles connecting to the iliac bone become tight and spasm. This causes pain. LOTS of pain! In fact all the nerves that make your entire leg and foot feel and move travel from your lower back, around the SIJ and through the hip. There are so many nerves in this area that if the bones are out of place there is a good chance that these nerves will get pinched. And you know what that means… pain traveling down your leg. SIJ pain can shoot into your back, groin, hip, leg or even foot. As with any time a nerve is pinched, you could also feel numbness, tingling, burning, coldness, heat or heaviness in the leg instead of pain. Many muscles connect to the iliac bone including muscles of the back, stomach, hips and gluteal region. Unfortunately, all these muscles are fair game for causing you pain.

Another common cause of SIJ pain/dysfunction is pregnancy. When you are pregnant there is a hormone called "Relaxin" that is released in your body. Relaxin does just what it sounds like it would… it relaxes the ligaments in your body. This is needed to allow the pelvis to expand to hold the baby. As the ligaments expand and stretch, they are less stable and more likely to be injured. Complications during labor can also cause your pelvis to shift during the delivery. This can include the baby having difficulty coming out of the birth canal, baby leaning on one side of your body more than the other, the doctor needing to manually extract the baby, back labor, or others. These things can place more force on one side of the pelvis more than the other and cause a shift. Relaxin is also present for another 2 weeks after the baby is born and/or the entire time you are breast feeding. So just because Junior is out of your body, doesn't mean you're out of the woods! The SIJ is delicate and easy to injure as long as the Relaxin is in your body.

Are you ready for the kicker??? SIJ Dysfunction will very rarely show up on an MRI. The MRI will show the bones, discs and nerves are intact and you will often be told there is nothing wrong. This can be very disheartening to people who have been in pain. It can make people feel like it's "all in their head". Many times it will only be a Physical Therapist that will be able to diagnose this issue after a thorough examination.

SIJ injuries can even pinch the nerves that control your bowels or bladder. Make sure to **see your doctor immediately if you notice loss of control of the bowel or bladder** as this could be the sign of something serious.

Signs of Sacro Iliac Joint Dysfunction (SIJ)

1. Pain is worse with sitting
    a. You may have to shift in your seat often in order to stay seated
2. Pain is worse with standing still
    a. Makes you to stand on one leg and kick the other leg to the side
    b. Shift weight from one side to the other as you stand
3. Pain is better with walking
4. Pain is worse with laying on your back, better laying on your side or belly.
5. Common when pregnant/ after giving birth.
6. Pain is usually lower in the back/buttock area.
7. Pain is usually slightly off to one side of the back and not directly in the center of the back.

Hands on or manual style physical therapy can help re-align your SI joint. By manually stretching, massaging and moving the bones of your spine and pelvis, your PT can help realign your SI joint ... without medication, shots or surgery! Physical therapy can then work on building your strength to support your spine. By strengthening the muscles that connect to the pelvis, the muscles will take the strain when you move. This will decrease the pressure on your SI Joint and other bones of the spine. This lets you move (or stay still) with little or no pain. What are you waiting for! Are you ready to "Heal Your Body, Live Your Life!" ??? Ask your PT about Hands-On or Manual PT today!

5

Postural

YOUR MOTHER ALWAYS used to tell you to sit up straight. Guess what?? She was right! Poor posture not only makes you slump forward, makes you look older than you are, but it can cause pain too! Your body is a wonderful machine. It can handle a lot. But like any other machine, it works best when the pieces are in the right place. If you use a machine with the parts out of place it will not work correctly. The same is true with your body. It is made to tolerate stress and activities with the spine in the correct posture. If you are hunched forward at your computer your spine is no longer working in the right spot. This places stress and strain on the wrong parts of the body. Continue this for years and years and it is no wonder you would have pain! When you slump forward repeatedly the muscles will become tight in this wrong position. It will make some muscles too tight (especially in your chest and the top of your neck) and some muscles weak (especially in your lower neck and upper back).

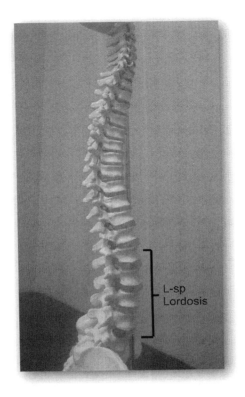

Signs of postural pain:

1. There was no injury, pain began "all of a sudden".
2. Pain is worse when you are still.
3. Pain improves with movement.
4. Ok, ok... you admit your posture stinks!

But I can't sit up straight, it hurts too bad!

If you have had poor posture for years, it will take a while to correct. Your body is used to the poor posture and that is what feels normal to you. The "right" posture doesn't even feel right. Usually this is because your muscles have tightened up in the wrong position.

When this happens you will need to work at stretching your muscles to allow your body to sit or stand up straight. The muscles in your neck, chest and upper back are usually the most problematic. A physical therapist can help identify which muscles you need to stretch, which muscles to you need to strengthen and how to get you standing up straight without making the pain worse.

By using the correct exercises and Hands-On, Manual style physical therapy, PT's can help you re-align your posture. This will allow your body to take pressure off of the overused areas and allow your body to function in its ideal position. Just like a machine, your body works the best when all the parts are in the right place. Once you can move better with less pain, we will focus on strengthening your core muscles. This will make sure your good posture stays and does not revert back to how it was before. Strengthening also helps pull you into your "good posture"... without even trying!

Extra Bonus

When you have good posture, not only will you feel better, but you will look better... and younger... and most likely taller!

Physical therapists specialize in how to do this without aggravating your pain... and doing it without medication, shots, or surgery!

So what are you waiting for? Are you ready to "Heal Your Body, Live Your Life!" ??? Ask your PT about Hands-on or Manual physical therapy today!

6

To FREEZE or NOT to FREEZE...
that is the question!

|HEAR THIS question every day... multiple times a day... "Do I use Ice or Heat on my back?"

This answer is complicated and will no doubted be longer than the one you were looking for. Ok, here we go...

In general, ICE is never wrong. When in doubt, use the ice. (I know, I hate ice too. But it works!)

Let's think of a car accident. Someone calls "911" and tells them "I've been in a car accident". Now the 911 operator is not there at the accident. They cannot fully assess the scenario over the phone and cannot be sure what emergency services will be required at the scene. So what happens? They send out the Ambulance, a few EMS workers, a Police car, maybe a 2nd police car and then a fire truck. Just in case. It's better to be safe than sorry.

Your body is the same way. Any time you get hurt, your body rushes various different things to the area to help you heal. It tends to send more things than needed, just in case. These things take up room and the injured area will start to swell. The swelling will build up in your joint and take up space. It will press on various different structures (bones, nerves, muscles, etc). This makes it more difficult to move the injured area. It also causes that "dull, achy, throbbing" pain. Ice stops the swelling. It both improves the swelling that is present and prevents swelling from beginning. So any time you injure yourself… the FASTER you can get ice on the area … the LESS swelling will occur… and the better you will feel.

ICE:

1. When you have a new injury
    a. Ie- If you lift up a box and feel a pull in your back.
2. Any time you have swelling
3. Apply immediately after the injury, or as soon as you can
4. If the injury or swelling persists more than a few days, SEE A HEALTH CARE PROFESSIONAL. Swelling means there is something wrong beneath the surface and continued swelling means the problem needs more than rest and ice to heal.

OK, so when do I use heat??

Heat helps to relax muscles. It will loosen the muscle fibers, relax spasms and decrease that tight feeling. Heat is good for more chronic injuries, or things that have been ongoing for more than 3 months. So if you have had a dull, pulling back pain for the past 3 years, heat will be your best option. Do you feel stiff and achy in the mornings? Heat will be great to put on your back when you wake up to loosen the muscles and help work out that morning stiffness. It is great for arthritis!

Moist heat is always the best. That means a hot shower, warm bath, hot tub, warm towel, etc. If you do not have moist heat, a regular hot pack will be fine. It is not moist heat, but will help loosen the muscles just the same. Every once in a while someone with chronic long standing pain will tell me that Ice works best for them. This is fine. As I said before, ice is never wrong. But when you CAN use heat, it is usually works better.

Heat should NOT be used when you have swelling. Heat works by bringing more blood flow to the area. This will make swelling worse! So it should NOT be used any time an area already has swelling. It may relax the area and feel good for a little bit, but by the next day the area will be more swollen, tight and achy.

Use HEAT for:

1. Chronic issues- present for over 3 months
2. Arthritis
3. Tight muscles
4. When NO swelling is present

When do I alternate hot and cold?

This answer is complex. It really takes the knowledge of a trained professional to know when to alternate ice and heat. Don't do this at home kids, talk to a PT first.

7

How do I know if I'm getting good treatment?

WHEN YOU ARE referred to physical therapy you can go to ANY physical therapy clinic. Even if your doctor has suggested or written down a certain location, you are the consumer and YOU can choose where you want to go. This is true for all insurance companies.

So knowing that YOU have the power... how do you choose where YOU want to go?

ANSWER: Do your research!

1. Ask your friends, family and neighbors for recommendations. You probably know someone who has been to physical therapy, whether they have mentioned going or not. Ask around. The reference from a trusted person in your life is always the most reassuring.

2. What is convenient for you? Is there a clinic close to your home or office? Does one clinic offer before or after work

appointments that will be easier to attend? Are there any other convenience factors one clinic has over another?

    a. For example, in my clinic we offer FREE Child Care for our patients during their appointments. We serve many military members who do not have family in the area. This helps many people attend therapy even if they do not have local family or friends to watch their children.

One BIG reason people do not get better in physical therapy is because it is difficult for them to attend appointments. Give yourself a fighting chance to succeed and make it as easy as possible to follow your therapist's advice.

3. Research the clinic you are thinking of attending. Go online and look at their webpage. What is their motto? What are their beliefs about health care and physical therapy? Do they only focus on one area of pain or do they take into account how the entire body works together? Do they ask you what YOUR goals are? It is important that PT focuses on what you want to return to and what lifestyle you want to regain. Make sure to go somewhere that is interested in what YOU think is important.

4. Tour the clinic. You are always allowed to go to a facility and ask for a tour of the gym and workout space. Make sure they have up-to-date equipment, attentive staff and a friendly atmosphere. You will be spending a good deal of time in PT and you want to be comfortable. You also want to make sure the facility has enough equipment to support your needs. A facility that does not allow you to take a tour or does not take the time to answer your questions may clue you into the fact that they may not have the welcoming and supportive environment you are looking for.

5. Research the physical therapists. Do they Specialize in any type of care? Are they Certified in any special techniques? The best therapists will believe in life-long learning. They will usually have gained various Specialties or Certifications throughout the years. Even if they do not specialize in your specific injury, Specializing shows they are up-to-date with their learning and provide current researched-based treatments. (ie- They can get you feeling BETTER QUICKER!)

8

Hands-On "Manual" Physical Therapy

THROUGHOUT MY YEARS practicing I have learned and experimented with many different methods of treating. I have found that by far, the best way to obtain significant, long-lasting results, is with Hands-On physical therapy.

As I explained earlier, when I started my Physical Therapy career I used stretching and strengthening exercises. This helped. I got 50% of my patients better. But what about the other 50% that did not get better? I decided that a 50% success rate was much lower than I wanted to offer my patients. My patients come to me for help because they cannot do the things they want to do. They cannot sleep, are unable to work, unable to take care of their children or grandchildren, unable to go to the gym... or even get out of bed by themselves! Telling half of them there was nothing that can be done seemed unacceptable.

Being a scientist, I began researching and testing different approaches. I started using a Hands-On therapy approach to some of my patients. I started adding massage to the sore muscles and tendons. I began manually stretching the stiff joints. I began working out the scar tissue. What did I notice?? My patients started to get better. Even the people with more difficult diagnoses responded well! So I continued. I continued my research, I continued my testing and I continued my learning. I added more Hands-On techniques until I was performing Hands-On Therapy to ALL of my patients. In fact, one of the main reasons I opened my own clinic was to ensure I could treat my patients the way I wanted to treat them… and using Hands-On therapy was one of them! There is something healing about putting your hands on someone's body. It allows you to truly feel the pain… you can identify the muscle tightness, knots or even weakness. With Hands-On Physical therapy, I can use my hands to feel exactly what is going on in the body… as well as my eyes to see.

As you can imagine using Hands-On therapy takes your PT extra time. In this day and age many places do not allow their PT's to take this extra time with their patients. Before signing up, always ask if the clinic believes in a "Hands-On" or "Manual" approach.

COMMON QUESTIONS:

1. **Q: How long is this going to take to go away?**
    A: It depends…it depends on YOU.

    In general, it takes to 4 to 8 weeks to go through the first 2 phases of healing (achieving no pain, all movement and strength returning to normal).

    It may take another 1 to 4 months to get back to all activities you want to do…depending on how active you are. This is the third phase of healing.

Here are 10 variables that determine how fast someone can heal:

- Overall health. Healthy people heal faster. Younger people heal faster.
- Other health issues such as diabetes, heart disease, high blood pressure, tobacco use, alcohol abuse and body weight all influence healing rates...and make the time to heal longer.
- Diet. People who consume more nutrients in their calories (Dr. Joel Fuhrman calls this "Nutrarian") heal faster than those who primarily eat processed foods.
- Rest levels. Our bodies need sleep and rest to rebuild. A lack of sleep slows healing time.
- Stress levels. People who have high levels of stress heal more slowly.
- Sedentary lifestyle. People who sit all day for work or to watch TV heal more slowly.
- People who follow advice and instruction from top level healthcare professionals heal more quickly than those who do not follow-through with care.
- People who are highly aware of their daily postures and habits heal more quickly...because they can adjust habits such as sleep or sitting positions more quickly.
- Readers heal more quickly. People with higher attention spans are more likely to be self-educated on a topic and more likely to follow-through with successful treatment.
- People who think there's hope tend to be more persistent and won't let anything stop them. (Recently we had a man with sciatica fly from Colorado to Pennsylvania to be successfully treated for sciatica).

2. **Q: How long before I see improvements?**

   A: Most people we see in the clinic see improvements within 1 to 2 weeks. If you go longer than 2 weeks without feeling better or moving better…you may be wrong about the cause of your sciatica regardless of what your X-ray or MRI shows.

3. **Q: Can I be completely healed or will this come back again?**

   A: Most people we see who *complete* the 3 Phases of Healing (meaning they no longer have pain, motion and strength are back to normal and they're back to doing all the activities they want to do without pain)…they have a minimal chance the pain will return.

   The stronger the person is…the less likely the sciatica symptoms will come back. This means you continue to do your therapy *not just until the pain goes away*, but until your body is strong enough to return to your previous activities.

   Your body is a bit like a car. If you take care of it, regularly change the oil and keep it running and fine tuned…there is little chance of break down.

   If you ignore it…very likely to break down and be in need of repair.

4. **Q: Which exercises should I do?**

   A: The best exercises for you depend on what the cause of your sciatica is.

DR. SARA S. MORRISON

We covered the 4 most common causes…
Herniated discs
Stenosis, arthritis
Pelvic or SI joint problem
Posture

Each has a series of gradually more advanced exercises.

So the key to picking the right exercise is to find the cause of your sciatica. Physical Therapists are Movement Specialists. They can help you with this.

5. **Q: How often should I do the exercises? And do I need to do them forever?**
   A: Most people we work with in the clinic for sciatica do the exercises at least once per day…every day.

Some will do them up to 3 times per day.

Doing the same exact exercises for years without changing could be a mistake.

In general, to get stronger, your exercise should progress and get more difficult.

With training your body adapts.

Keeping that in mind, there are 2 rules to training:

1. Everything works.
2. Nothing works forever.

This means that any exercise (although painful) may make you stronger.

But once your body adapts, it's time to move on to something different or more challenging.

One of the best programs you can move on to once you complete the 3 Phases of Healing for your Sciatica is a consistent walking program.

People who walk every day have less risk of reinjuring their back and sciatica.

6. Q: What do I need to do for complete care? Am I going to relapse?
    A: The best thing to do for sciatica, if you are worried about it coming back again in the future, is to complete all 3 phases of healing.

    Phase One is where you focus on getting rid of the pain, numbness and tingling.

    Phase Two is where you focus on getting normal movement back and full strength.

    Phase Three is where you go back to previous activities you want to do.

    In our clinic, after we see a person who had sciatica…and they are now pain free and have full motion and full strength, we ask:

    "What activities have you avoided in the past month that you want to get back to doing?"

Some will say walking, or golfing or gardening...something along those lines.

And we'll tell that person to begin to ad those activities to their normal routine. That way we can make sure they are truly strong enough to "get back to normal".

They keep doing their exercises at home to get stronger and stronger.

Most come back for a recheck appointment in 2 months and have no trouble at all.

Some do have a relapse.

We then take a look at the activity and at the program and help them get on the right track.

As mentioned before, people who are stronger recover more quickly...

So it's usually only one or two visits before that person is on the right track again.

7. **Q: Which position should I sleep in?**
   A: On your back is best.

   Next would be on your side.

   Last would be on your stomach.

Regardless, an important key is to keep your spine in "neu-tral". This means that it is not twisted to the right or left... but keeps the natural curve it normally has.

Pillows of folded towels can be placed under your knees, under your side, or under your feet to help you sleep in the least painful position for you.

9

Do I need any special equipment?

A : AT TOTAL Body Therapy & Wellness we have state-of-the-art equipment. We keep our technology on the cutting edge to ensure that our patients get the best treatments available.

This includes:

1. Cold Laser Therapy
2. Total Body Vibration
3. Traction
4. BIODEX Balance System
5. Spinal Manipulation
6. Dry Needling

In conjunction with your treatments in the clinic, you will be given exercises that can be done at home with a simple ball, exercise bands and a safe place to exercise.

Cold Laser Therapy

Cold Laser Therapy (or CLT) is an extremely effective way to manage pain and accelerate the healing process in new and pre-existing injuries. This helps reduce or completely eliminate pain, decrease swelling or inflammation and accelerate tissue healing by rates **up to 40 percent.** The best part about CLT is that it is safe for everyone!

CLT is different from other forms of treatment in that it works on the cellular level to promote the stimulation of chemical reactions within the cells themselves. CLT is similar to photosynthesis in plants (Remember Biology class? The light from the sun stimulates the plant cells to grow) Light is absorbed by the body and converted into energy that the body can use for growth.

How does it increase cell function?

1. Increased and accelerated healing of soft tissue and bone.
2. Increases T-Cell production (the healing cells of the body) which support immune function.
3. Increased production of Neurotransmitters which improve nerve function.

Total Body Vibration

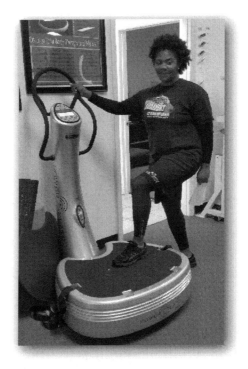

Total Body Therapy & Wellness' Total Body Vibration machine is ideal to stretch or strengthen any muscle. It uses a combination of amplitude and frequency to cause an impulse in the targeted muscles forcing them to involuntarily contract. This causes rapid contraction and relaxation of muscles at 25 to 50 times per second. This means it will cause your muscles to work really hard the entire time you are on it.

I like to think of it as an Electric Physio Ball. When you sit on a physioball, even if you are just sitting there, your back and abdominal muscles are activating to keep you balanced. You do not feel tired, but they are working hard. Our TBV does the same thing, except it vibrates much faster and causes the muscles to work much harder than the physioball does. So even if you just stand on the TBV, you are strengthening your muscles and burning calories! They best part is, it's not hard! You barely feel yourself working. Now the next day may be a different story, but it allows you to strengthen and stabilize your muscles faster and without pain.

The TBV is GREAT for swelling! It works as a pump on both the circulatory and lymphatic systems. It increases the speed of blood flow and lymphatic drainage throughout the body. This rapidly increases strength, stability, range of motion and pumps out swelling FASTER than any other stability ball or machine! It's also great for anyone with Peripheral Neuropathy or Diabetes!

Lumbar Traction

Spinal traction is a form of decompression therapy that relieves pressure on the spine. It can be performed manually or mechanically. Spinal traction is used to treat herniated discs, sciatica, degenerative disc disease, pinched nerves, and many other back conditions.

Spinal traction stretches the spine to take pressure off compressed discs. It causes a vacuum or "negative pressure" that sucks the disc back into place... or puts the jelly back into your donut. This will take pressure off the nerves and reduce the pain shooting down the leg. Traction also straightens the spine and stretches the muscles of the back and pelvis. Many people have avoided back surgery with the use of traction! It doesn't hurt (it actually feels great) and takes only 15-20 minutes.

PS- There is a traction for neck pain and headaches too!

Candidates

People with pain in the back and down the leg. It is most commonly used to treat bulging discs, degenerative disc disease, herniated discs, facet disease, sciatica, foraminal stenosis, sacro-iliac pain and pinched nerves.

BIODEX Balance System

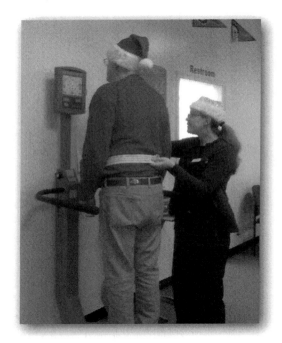

Balance is my passion. My love. 1 out of 3 Senior Citizens falls every year. I aim to stop this

Here's how:

Total Body Therapy & Wellness utilizes the **Biodex Balance System** in order to test, analyze and improve stability and balance of our patients.

The Biodex benefits all patients with mobility and balance difficulties as well as patients suffering from Vertigo or after a leg injury or surgery. All patients of Total Body Therapy and Wellness benefit from this therapy tool in order to improve overall strength, stability and balance. Biodex provides objective data (numbers) for insurance companies so they can see your improvement. This also serves as great input and motivation for patients... especially if you have a stubborn family member that thinks their "balance is fine".

Benefits of BIODEX Balance System:

1. Easy to understand information for patients
2. Helps stubborn family members realize their problem
3. Accurate balance testing to see if you are safen
4. Objective Data for your Doctor and Insurance Compay
5. Pinpoints your weakest area for your PT

How does it work?

The screen of the Biodex will show a picture. Your body is represented by a black dot. The black dot will move when you move. If you lean left, the dot moves left. Each test or "game" on the Biodex will instruct you to do a certain activity. You will either have to maintain your body as still as possible or lean towards a certain blinking target. The black dot will move as you move and trace a line showing you where you leaned. Sometimes this line is straight, showing you moved in a controlled manner. Sometimes this line is squiggly, showing you moved in an unbalanced way. Basically, the closer your screen resembles the drawing your 5 year old Granddaughter drew for you, the more unsteady your balance is!

The Biodex will provide a picture of your balance as well as a score. The balance system will score your balance based on the percent of time you were steady vs the percent of time you were unsteady. This picture can be printed off and sent to your Doctor or Insurance company to show them where your balance started and how it has improved with physical therapy.

I.E.- if you score a 40/100 that means 40% of the time you were moving you were controlled and balanced. 60% of the time you were UNBALANED or Falling.

It is also great information for your PT! As you lean different directions, not only will you get an overall Balance Score, but you will get a score for each of 9 different directions (leaning forward, right, backwards, backwards on the left, forwards on the right, etc). This shows your PT which direction you favor and which direction you have the most difficulty with. The PT can then customize your treatment to improve what you have specific problems with.

The goal is to bring your balance to at least 65% in all directions. If your balance is at least 65% there is a high chance that you will regain your balance and not fall if you slip. If it is less than 65%, you a considered at a high risk of falling. Your body will most likely not be able to regain control if you lose your balance. By practicing on the Biodex System you will train your body to react faster when you lose your balance and how to return your body's center of gravity to normal.

- Faster reaction time will help you avoid obstacles and keep yourself upright if you start to fall. Improved coordination can help prevent falls

- Stronger muscles and bones can buffer the impact of a fall and make your body more resistant to fractures
- Better brain function. Regular exercise helps maintain brain function with age. Clearer thinking may help you avoid situations that increase fall risk.

The Biodex Balance System has several training modules to help maintain and improve balance over time. These include:

- Postural Stability Training - helps train your body to maintain ideal posture and static standing balance (standing still). The screen looks like a target or a "Bulls Eye". Your body is represented by a black dot. You need to keep the dot in the center of the target.
- Limits of Stability- This trains your moving or Dynamic Balance. The LOS trains your body in moving in one direction and then bringing yourself back to neutral. This simulates you losing your balance and falling. It will train your body how to bring yourself back to neutral after a loss of balance.
- Maze Control Training - improves your body's motor control and coordination skills
- Weight Shift Training - trains the body to find/hold its center of gravity in various positions which is excellent for orthopaedic/joint injuries. Shows if you are still favoring your "bad side".

People that are considered "Higher Risk for Falls", include but not limited to people with:

- Parkinson's
- Stroke or other Cardiac Issues

- After surgery- including hip or knee replacement
- Vertigo
- Multiple Sclerosis
- Cancer patients
- anyone that has been on bed rest or stayed in the hospital
- Deconditioned older adults

Studies show that balance, strength, and flexibility training not only improve walking, but also help reduce the risk of falling

Spinal Manipulation

Spinal manipulation, also called spinal manipulative therapy, is designed to relieve pressure on joints, reduce inflammation, and improve movement between bones. It's often used to treat back, neck and headache pain.   In **spinal manipulation**, the therapist uses their hands to apply a controlled, sudden force to a specific joint.

For this technique the physical therapist will apply a short, quick thrust over restricted joints (one at a time) with the goal of restoring normal range of motion in the joint. The patient's body is positioned in specific ways to optimize the adjustment of the spine. Patients often hear popping noises, like when you crack your knuckles. This technique will usually provide immediate decrease in pain! (yay!) It is only temporary (boo!) so it NEEDS TO BE COMBINED WITH EXERCISE to make the effects last. Spinal Manipulation will allow your bones to move better, decrease your pain and increase your motion. You can then strengthen the muscles with the spine correctly aligned.

Some people should avoid spinal manipulation or adjustments, including people who have severe osteoporosis, high stroke risk, spinal cancer, have metal in the spine or an unstable spine. People who experience numbness, tingling, or loss of strength in an arm or leg should also avoid these treatments.

10

Dry Needling

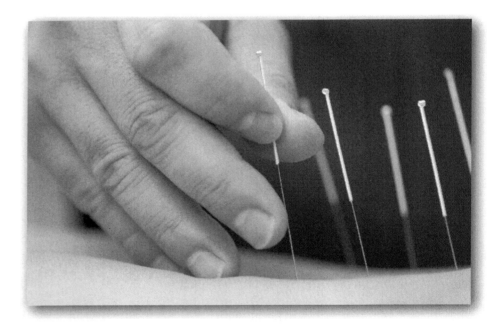

What is dry needling?

Dry needling uses a very small needle, similar to a sewing needle. It looks like an acupuncture needle, except longer. They are considered "dry" because they do not inject medication or fluid into the body. Since they are not hollow, like injection needles, they are a smaller circumference or "gauge". Standard flu shot needles are 13 to 14 gauge needles. The Dry Needles are 0.15 mm to 0.33 mm in circumference. This is roughly 39 times smaller than standard flu shot needs. In other words, they are SUPER TINY! These tiny needles are inserted through the skin and directly into the muscles, scar tissue, or tendons below. Once the needles are inserted in the skin they are manipulated or twisted and grab onto muscle knots and scar tissue. They are left in the skin for a certain time period and then removed. During this time, the muscle knotting and scar tissue is physically broken up.

How do muscles normally work?

Muscles are made up of many small muscle fibers. These fibers are parallel and glide and slide along each other as a muscle contracts and relaxes. When the muscles are over worked, strained or injured, they become knotted up. Just like a bunch of necklaces that you put in a case, they can tangle around each other. When the fibers are knotted or tangled, they can no longer slide and slide along each other. This causes pain or inability to use a muscle when your body tries to contract it.

These muscles knots are identified by your therapist and dry needles are inserted into them. When the needles are twisted, the abnormal fibers wrap around the needle. Your therapist can tell they are wrapping around the needle because it takes more force to turn the needle. The needle is turned until the patient experiences a spreading sensation.

Many times the muscles are so knotted and tight that there is little blood flow to the area. This can make the area numb. In this case, the needles are twisted until the tissue is wound around them so much that they will no longer turn.

DR. SARA S. MORRISON

When all the needles are inserted and twisted, the patient is left in this position until they are removed. In my clinic, we usually leave them in the skin for 10 minutes on the first day and 15 to 20 minutes on the following treatments. Needles can be left in the body for up to 45 minutes. During that time the patient remains still, as moving with needles inserted into muscle could cause pain.

How do the dry needles release the muscle knots?

Initially when you are hurt, your body tries very hard to fix the injury. In an "all hands on deck" mode, it sends everything is can to the area to help fix it. This is why after you stub your toe, the area becomes very red and swollen. Blood and cells are rushing to the area to fix the pain. This is called the Acute phase of healing and is the most painful. This lasts about 3 months. After this 3 month mark, your body moves into the Chronic Phase. During this phase the body becomes accustomed to the pain. It thinks "Ok guys, this is how we are now. We will have to learn to deal with it."

As pain becomes chronic, the body is not trying very hard to fix it and instead tries to manage it. Your body realizes that it cannot tolerate this strong pain forever and "gets used to it". Often people will tell me that they cannot give their pain a number on a scale of 0-10. Patients will often say "I'm just used to it now, I try not to think about it" or "It's a 5/10 to me, but to anyone else it would be a 10/10."

During the chronic phase the body is now accustomed to pain and thinks of it as the "new normal". This is how we are now. The spine will send altered signals to the muscles telling them it is now normal to be knotted. When dry needles are inserted and wrap the muscle fibers around them it resets the signal.

I like to think of it as rebooting a computer. We all have been us-ing our computers when all of a sudden something just isn't work-ing right. Maybe your email won't send or your favorite website won't open up. So what do we do? We restart the computer. When it reboots everything back up, it goes back to normal settings and everything works right.

Dry needling works in the same way to reset the signal form the spine to the muscle. It stops the abnormal message from the spine that tells the muscle "this knotted painful position is how we are supposed to be now" and it allows it to resend its original signal saying "RELAX" to the muscle. As the procedure is repeated, it re-inforces the message and breaks up the altered message to various different muscles.

As with anything, the longer your pain has been present and the stronger the muscle knotting is, the more treatments you will need. Dry needling treatments can go from 1 to 15 sessions per area.

What is Dry Needling good for?
Dry needling is good for chronic conditions, or anything that has been bothering you for longer than 3 months. It works with many conditions such as: muscle knotting, muscles spasms, tendonitis, migraines/headaches, carpal tunnel, plantar fasciitis, Golfer's el-bow/Tennis elbow or epicondylitis, and many other conditions. It can also remove scar tissue surrounding nerves and improve the functioning of the nerve.

Dry needling will break up muscle knotting or spasms and break up scar tissue. This includes myofascial conditions. The myofascial is a thin layer of tissue between the muscles and the skin. It is similar to that whitish film that coats raw chicken breasts. The tissue cov-ers all the muscles in your entire body from head to toe. Because it covers the entire body Myofascia tightness in one area can cause pain in a completely different area. This is the main cause of pain in multiple areas with myofascial conditions such as Fibromyalgia (FMS).

When can Dry Needling NOT be used?

1. If you are taking blood thinners. Taking an aspirin a day is fine, but if you are on medications that drastically thin you blood (i.e Coumadin) you may bleed excessively when the needles are removed. That would be bad. We are not prepared for people bleeding excessively in an outpatient setting and therefore will not perform dry needling on these patients.

2. If you are taking antibiotics. If you are taking antibiotics that means that there is an infection in your body. We do not want to introduce a new substance inside the body that will potentially disrupt your healing process. Dry needling can be initiated several days after your antibiotic course is finished.

3. If your condition is in the Acute Phase of healing (less than 3 months old). During the Acute Phase of healing, your body is actively trying its best to heal your injury. Your body is always the best healer. We let your body heal itself for the first 3 months. If your pain persists after 3 months, dry needling can be initiated.

Precautions:

If you have any of these conditions, your therapist will discuss these issues with you. Dry needling may or may not be appropriate for you based on details of your specific condition.

1. Seizures

   Seizures can cause your body to shake uncontrollably. If you have a seizure with the needles inside your body this could be dangerous as the needles could injure your body. If you have a history of seizures you will need to discuss when, why, and how often they occur with your therapist.

2. Sensitivity to metal

   The needles are metal. If you are sensitive to metal, this could aggravate your skin. So we don't do it. (This one should be obvious).

3. Diabetic or altered skin

   If you have altered sensation you may not be able to feel the needles and may not be able to feel if they cause you unusual pain.

4. History of fainting

   Just like seizures, we don't want you fainting during the dry needling procedure. Your history of fainting, including when, why, and how often they occur, will be discussed with your therapist.

Important To Remember

Dry needing is a specialty of physical therapy. It requires extensive training, beyond the 7 years in PT school, to become a **Certified Dry Needling PT**. NOT ALL Physical Therapists are able to perform Dry Needling.

How do I find a good Physical Therapy Clinic?

When looking for a Physical Therapy clinic, ask if they have PT's that are certified in Dry Needling. If they are dry needling certified that means they have extensive experience in working with muscle spasms and chronic pain. Even if dry needling is not right for you, a Certified Dry Needling PT will be sure to know many techniques that will work for chronic pain.

Dry Needling Success Story

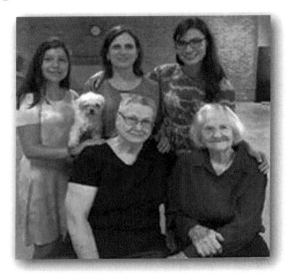

"I AM PAM Jonas and I have been going to Total Body Therapy And Wellness Clinic this past year for excruciating chronic neck, back and shoulder pain along with fibromyalgia. It was during my work as a Labor and Delivery nurse for over 25 years, I had undergone multiple low back surgeries as well a rotator cuff repair. After the last three level lumbar fusion in 2006, I had to learn how to walk again and unfortunately was determined disabled. It was my faith in God and my supportive family that helped me to keep strong as I struggled in and out of many doctors offices and physical therapy places trying to find ways to cope with my miserable state of being.

It wasn't until I finally remembered a place years earlier that I took my youngest daughter to for her physical therapy at TBT&W, that I thought I would try it for myself. From first day I hobbled into the TBT&W clinic until now, I have been transformed! I have virtually been bedridden since 2006 and now I can walk upright and partici-pate in my girls' lives!

The moment Dr. Sara Morrison spoke to me and placed her hands on me, I just knew it was the Lord that brought me there. From that day on, I have received the most compassionate and professional care by each member of TBT&W team. I can't say enough about the help and the progress that I have made from an intervention called Dry Needling.

Dry Needling is a form of physical therapy that involves inserting a very thin acupuncture needle through the skin and into a trigger point muscle. The trigger point is stimulated by the needle to se-crete chemicals to bathe the area of inflammation and pain. Within minutes, the muscle resets itself to its normal state. CURED".

11

Top 3 Reasons Not To Attend Pt

1. **I don't have enough time.**
   1. I don't buy this excuse! When most people rate their priorities, "health" is high on the list. Yet when it comes to their medical appointments they cannot make the time. This is about your back. You only have one (and to my knowledge, they haven't figured out how to replace those yet!) This is about you returning to the activities you enjoy. This is about you taking control of your life instead of the pain controlling you. Many of my patients have busy lives. I have treated Business Owners, Mothers of small children, people with no cars, people with two jobs and people who were told by their doctors they would never walk again. They are all busy, yet they all made the time. Their back was a priority to them. So like I said…I'm not buying it. Make the time.

2. **I have a high copay/ I don't have Health Insurance**
   Physical Therapy has been found to be much more effective and less costly than other interventions (Medication, Injections, Surgery, etc). Add up the costs you are already incurring due to your pain:

i.   Extra time out of work
ii. Medications- both prescription and over the counter
iii. Hiring additional child care

Then think about the things you cannot put a price on:

iv. Missing activities with your family
v.   Losing sleep
vi. Less productive when you hurt or did not sleep well
vii. Your job is mad because of your missed work
viii. You are not able to do the things you enjoy

It will cost you less in the long run to heal your pain with PT. In my clinic, Total Body Therapy & Wellness, we offer payment plans as well as Private Pay rates for those without insurance. We also give you a customized Home Exercise Program to do at home. Performing this exactly as your PT instructs will limit the amount of visits you will need to make. Ask if these services are available at your local clinic.

3. I have tried PT in the past and it didn't work.
I have 2 questions for you:
1. Did you follow your therapist's orders?
   i.   Did you perform your exercises as often as you were sup- posed to?
   ii. Did you attend physical therapy as instructed?
   iii. Did you limit your activities at home and work and avoid "over doing it"?
        Just like you can't blame the car for breaking down if you don't change the oil… you can't blame the physical therapy for "not working" if you don't do it as instructed.
2. Did you receive "hands on" Physical Therapy?
   As I mentioned before, I have tried various kinds of physical therapy. Using hands on or manual style physical therapy, in

conjunction with stretching and strengthening the muscles, is the key. Without it, pain levels will remain higher. By using a hands-on or manual style approach you will note great improvement in the movement of the bones, the improvement in muscle knots and your overall pain levels. The PT can physically:

1. Work out tightness in muscles
2. Break up scar tissue
3. Break up muscle knotting
4. Reduce swelling
5. Improve the movement in the joints/bones

If you did not have a Hands-On or Manual Style approach in your PT, you did not receive all the pieces. If you are looking for pain relief that is not medication, shots or surgery ... try it again with a clinic who practices this way.

12

Patient Testimonials

Don't take my word for it... listen to them!

"**A**FTER HAVING MY son, I had a difficult time at the end of the day. My back and neck were tired and I had a hard time falling asleep because my back was uncomfortable. Now, at the end of the day, I feel great! My back feels great ad I have enough energy to do my daily exercises and more! Taking care of my son is much easier after my therapy. He is growing everyday and picking him up and playing with him is fun instead of painful! Thank y'all for the help and strength!"
— *Holly Bradshaw, 32 years old, SIJ Dysfunction*

"I came to TBTW for sciatic nerve pain. Before coming to physical therapy I had difficulty bending, kneeling, walking, standing, working, and climbing stairs. I was in constant pain. At 44 years old, I was unsure what to do about my sciatic nerve pain. I felt I was too young to be having these issues. After multiple trips to various doctors, I had assumed I would have to live with this pain for the rest of my life and possibly have to have medication to cope with

the pain. I attended a lunch & learn about sciatic nerve pain hosted by Sara Morrison from TBTW and quickly made an appointment. Through stretching and exercise, they taught me at TBTW, I am now pain free and able to enjoy life again! I can do all the things that I was struggling with before I started therapy and am completely pain free! Sara and her staff are the best!"
— *Paul Thomas, 42 years old, Lower back and Sciatica pain*

"TBTW has been great! When I first started coming, I was having back and hip pain from an old injury sustained while I was in the Air Force. With their help and expertise, I have gotten a lot back that was lost due to the injury. They have been friendly, welcoming, understanding, and have pushed me when I needed it. Great customer service and friendly staff makes for a great experience! Thanks!"
— *Kristin Foley, 39 year old, lower back and hip pain*

"I went to Total Body Therapy & Wellness when I had back pain. Due to arthritis in my lower back it was hard for me to do all the normal things in life, and it even woke me at night. Like running and playing with my grandchildren. It would even bother me to walk, or stand for long periods of time. Sara Morrison and her team at Total Body helped me withtreatment and exercise. They even gave me some exercises to do at home, which I continue to do today!

I am now able to do the things I enjoy, and can play with my grandchildren without worrying about back pain. The Folks are Total Body Therapy & Wellness are wonderful. They are very knowledgeable and are very devoted to their patients. You're not just a number when you walk into their facility. They treat you like you're

part if their family. I highly recommend Total Body Therapy & Wellness to anyone who needs any kind of Physical Therapy".
— *Merrianne Chapman, 50 years old, DDD*

"I have been to TBTW twice for 2 different events in my life. In January 2015 I was hit head on at a very high rate of speed by a drunk driver. Miraculously, we both lived! I did not have any serious injuries but I was bruised and sore all over. I had pain in my right lower back that would not go away. I am a nurse, but despite years of patient care, never had any back pain. I did however have chronic hip pain for nearly 28 years. I had been to many doctors but none of them could find a cause. TBTW targeted my therapy plan for my low back pain AND in doing so they cured my hip pain I had for so many years! It has now been over 1 year since I finished therapy for my lower back and my low back pain AND hip pain have been totally gone! I returned to TBTW in June of 2016 after a rear-end accident caused whip lash pain to my neck and upper back. This too was something new – I had never had neck pain in the past. The pain was at the base of my head, down my neck and into my clavicle. I had a kink in my upper back. At work, my upper back ached and tired so easily. The TBTW staff again targeted the treatment for the areas that hurt and taught me how to do the exercises at home. I am now pain free once again! I am back at work & the kink is out of my back, the achiness and tiredness is gone! I am sleeping well without waking up from back/neck pain! TBTW is so wonderful and amazing!"
— *Pamela Cork, 44 years old, Lower Back/Hip Pain*

"Great Place. Came in with constant pain in the back. Unable to stand for long periods of time. The smallest task could bring my back pain

back. After 3 months and a lot of core exercises, I am able to work out in the gym again and take the dog for walks. TBTW has changed my life! Thank you!"
— *Raymond Stone, 45 years old, SIJ Pain*

"I came to physical therapy because of a car accident. I was having difficulties working out and doing much of anything without feeling pain. After physical therapy, I am now back in the gym! I am almost back to my normal self, prior to the car accident. Physical therapy has helped me strengthen my neck, shoulder, and back to the point where I can now go to the gym 3 to 4 times per week. As a former fitness competitor, physical therapy has put me back on track to where I could potentially compete in the next year! Recovery takes time and slow and steady always wins the race!"
— *Skyler Spinler, 34 years old, SIJ pain*

"Before therapy I had trouble bending and standing for long periods of time. Now I can walk longer and stand without pain. Physical therapy at TBTW was excellent. The staff never pushed me to do anything that caused pain. It greatly improved my ability to go back to the way I was. The staff was very nice and always smiling. They made me feel very welcome. I would highly recommend TBTW to everyone".
— *Eileen Cameron, 54 years old, DDD*

"I had sciatic pain on my right side (leg). My pain is totally gone. I really appreciate the therapists here at Total Body Therapy. Thank you for the expertise and great care. Definitely a total experience."
— *Anthony Lewis, 50 years old, Sciatica*

About the Author

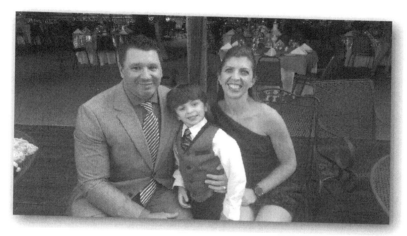

Dr. Sara S. Morrison

I HAVE BEEN A physical therapist in Harnett County since 2002. I received my Bachelors of Physical Therapy degree from the University at Buffalo of New York State and Doctorate of Physical Therapy from Arcadia University. In 2008 I opened Total Body Therapy & Wellness in Lillington, NC. The goal of this was to provide exceptional "Big City Care" in a small-town community.

I have been invited to speak on health and wellness issues in many areas of our community. In 2010 I received "Lillington Chamber of Commerce's Small Business of the Year" Award. I also served on Lillington Chamber of Commerce Board of Directors for 3 years and was President of Lillington Chamber of Commerce in 2013. As a way to give back to my profession, I mentor future physical therapists and other health care providers from many local colleges including Campbell University, University of North Carolina, Methodist University, Wake Technical College, and Western Carolina University. I also perform interviews at Campbell University's Doctorate of Physical Therapy School to select incoming students. My passion is to improve the quality of life for those in my community and to bring quality health care to rural settings.

When I am not working, I love to spend as much time as possible with my family! I love them so much I put their picture above! My husband Erik, son Blake and dogs Bella and Ellie (the dogs weren't invited to that wedding). I also enjoy running, reading, baking, sewing, watching football and going to the beach.

Throughout my career, I have specialized in many areas of health and wellness and have developed my own custom programs to treat many afflictions including:

Lower Back Pain, Lymphedema, Vertigo, Foot Pain, Pediatrics, Fall Prevention, TMJ and Headaches/Migraines.

I have become certified in many aspects of Physical Therapy including:

Certified Dry Needling
Functional Movement Taping
Certified Decongestive Therapist
Certified Functional Capacity Evaluator
Certified Fitter of Lymphedema Garments
Certified Neuro-Developmental Therapist of Children and Babies
Neuro-Anatomy of Developmental Pathologies

Made in the USA
Middletown, DE
27 May 2017